THE RE
CARLGIVER

THE RELUCTANT CAREGIVER

MAKING PEACE WITH AN IMPERFECT PARENT

KAREN OKE

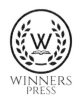

WINNERS
PRESS

Published in the United States by Winners Press, an imprint of
Winners LLC, winnerspress.com.

ISBN: 978-0-9712240-6-3

Printed in the United States of America

To my Best Friend, for staying with me in the dark and walking with me in the light. You are my life, my air, my all.
And to every caregiver who cleaned up, lifted up, picked up, washed up, cooked up, drove up, helped up, signed up, paid up, and listened up, even when you were fed up.

CONTENTS

THE RELUCTANT CAREGIVER

INTRODUCTION

"An unresolved issue will be like a cancer with the potential to spread into other areas of your relationship, eroding the joy, lightness, love, and beauty." — Liz Mullinar

Vanessa spent most of her time locked in her room to protect herself from her mother. Her mom had always been a demanding person. She was self-absorbed and depended on her daughter to fill in the gaps for what she lacked in herself and missed in the husband who had left her. Whether out of fear, selfishness, or some other dysfunction, her mother never seemed to care that Vanessa had no life of her own.

Like most young women, Vanessa wanted to find love, get married, and have children of her own, but she couldn't bring herself to leave her mom. Being an only child, in her mind, she was all her mother had. By the time she eventually started to consider striking out on her own, she was forced to stay.

Vanessa's mom was diagnosed with early-onset dementia. The thought of committing her mother to a state-run nursing home left Vanessa feeling she had no other choice but to step into the role of primary care-giver. For Vanessa, it was nothing short of a life sentence. As the dementia progressed, it caused her mom to become verbally and physically aggressive to the point where she would do physical harm to her own daughter.

Vanessa found herself trapped in a life she did not want but from which she saw no escape. She thought of herself as a dutiful daughter, but what she interpreted as duty was really taking on her mother's dysfunction. She had locked herself into a destructive pattern of enable-ment that left her depressed, bitter, and guilt-ridden.

Feelings of resentment towards her mother caused a series of stress-induced illnesses that proved detrimental to her overall health. Then Vanessa's mother died, leaving her a house filled with painful memories and a heart full of resentment. A year later, Vanessa met the love of her life and was planning to get married, but she never got to realize her dream. Vanessa, a beautiful, vibrant woman with no known illnesses before becoming a caregiver, died of ovarian cancer at thirty-one.

HOW AND WHY I WROTE THIS BOOK

I've been a psychotherapist for nearly two decades. I spend most of my days listening to people facing mental or emotional challenges and helping them cope with difficult situations. When I chose that career path, I had no idea that working through the issues of my own life and experiences with my mother would be what qualified me the most for that position.

My mother never went out of her way to give me the good parts of herself. For most of my life, she was either absent or dependent on me in ways that made me wish she was absent. Everything about the way she treated me shaped the decisions I made in life and carved out my insecurities. It took me years to realize that her deficiencies do not define me, and her issues don't have to be mine.

For a long time, I felt guilty about not having what I considered to be a normal close bond with my mother. *Loving. Considerate. Encouraging. Supportive. Positive. Affirming. Affectionate. Giving. Unselfish.* These were not words that I would have used to describe her. That is not a malicious statement. That's simply the truth, and I know that is not unique to me.

The reality is that there are many mothers for whom such descriptions are just not true. Some people have all-out anxiety attacks every year when Mother's Day approaches. I have met people whose mothers have died, and tears still come to their eyes when they speak of them. Their tears are not because of any fond remembrances, but because of the hurt, pain, and resentment that they are still dealing with as a result of having the mother they had. Then there are those who spent a good part of their lives neglected, abandoned, unloved, even abused, who find themselves in a position where they have to take care of a parent who did not or could not take care of them.

Caregiving is like a mirror that reflects your past, present, and future. It's a conversation, sometimes an argument, between the person you are because of your parent's past and the person you want to be. What makes this dialogue even more difficult is it may involve a parent who, though they created this conflict, may no longer be capable of helping you resolve it.

Whether you became a caregiver out of a sense of duty, obligation, or by default because there was no one else to do it, it is no easy task to deal with the day-to-day demands of taking care of someone else. Add to that the dichotomy of having to serve and sacrifice for a parent whose very presence has been associated with stress, chaos, and everything you're trying to avoid, and you have a scenario that's fraught with conflict. Just because a parent needs care, does not negate or erase their hurtful actions of the past. On the contrary, it intensifies them and drudges up painful memories. This book addresses the dilemma that is unique to those who are or were care-givers for a parent with whom they still have issues.

HOW THIS BOOK WILL BENEFIT YOU

When you board a flight, right before takeoff, the inflight attendant will make an announcement regarding various safety procedures. This announcement communicates pertinent information, especially for those who are accompanying someone who requires assistance. The attendant advises you to familiarize yourself with the aircraft and locate your nearest exit, keeping in mind that it may be behind you. It is recommended that you keep your seatbelt fastened at all times just in case there is unexpected turbulence. A critical portion of the announcement tells you to be sure to place the oxygen mask over your own mouth and nose before assisting others. This is usually the last thing a caregiver thinks of doing.

When you become a caregiver to a parent with whom you are in conflict, it's a lot like taking a flight in bad weather to an unknown destination. When you first board the plane, you may look around to try to familiarize yourself with your surroundings and find there is no exit sign behind you. Because of your location in the aircraft, when turbulence hits, you are likely to feel it the most, and the need to always be strapped in place ready to assist can feel forced and uncomfortable.

This book will point out some exit signs you may not have been able to see before now. It will show you ways you can adjust your emotional seatbelt so that you can be as comfortable as possible under the given circumstances. And it will serve as your oxygen mask so that you can preserve the life you should have instead of sacrificing it to the pain of your past or the pressure of your present responsibilities.

Writing this book was therapeutic for me. And although my story may be much different from yours, the process of taking an honest look at the way life was and is, then excavating and preserving those things that prove valuable moving forward is universal. I cannot say that my path to peace has been a smooth one. It was replete with frustration, but the lessons I learned have given me an advantage in any adverse situation, an advantage I want you to have.

As you read each chapter, there will be relevant principles that you can apply to your own life that will not only assist you in your role as a caregiver, but more importantly, your role in taking care of yourself. And now, I invite you into my story, not as an observer, but as a fellow comrade on this journey to peace.

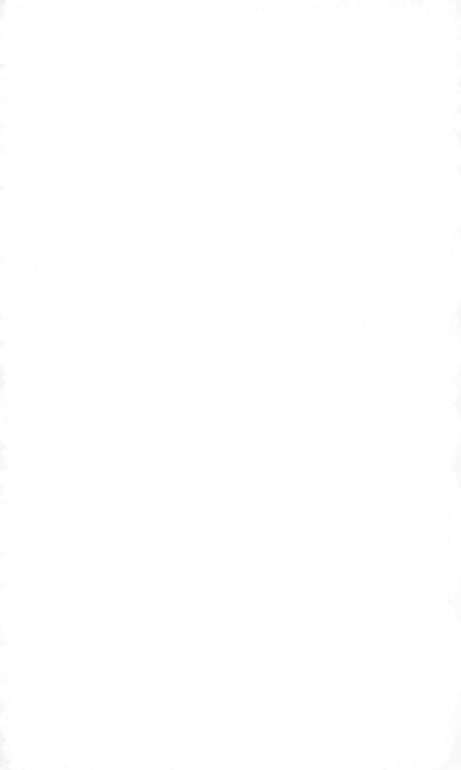

THE ACCIDENTAL DAUGHTER

My mum introduced me to God at a very young age. She left me for Him. The first time was when I was around four years old. She went to find the will of God in the sacred halls of a Bible school, 6,689 miles away from where I was born. Apparently, God's will for her had nothing to do with me.

I didn't know what to make of God in the beginning. He always seemed to be involved with my mother's drama which made Him suspect. Every time I got left behind, God was somehow involved. At least, that was my mother's version of the story. The preface to her leaving was always, "God told me ..." For a long time, I was never sure if God really told her these things or if she just didn't have enough courage to admit she did not want to stay. After all, God is the perfect scapegoat. You can blame Him for everything, and you know He is never going to defend Himself. God was very convenient.

I was born in Benin City, Nigeria, into a household that was as tumultuous as the country's political climate. My father was a drunkard and abusive in every sense of the word. I know who he is, but I have no relationship with him. Mum had a rough time getting pregnant. She tried for years. So, when she had me, it was kind of like a miracle.

When I was born, mum made up her mind that she didn't want any more kids. I'm sure she wanted me, or she wouldn't have kept trying. At least that's what I choose to believe. But I don't think motherhood was quite what she expected.

She gave me the name Karen. I found out later that it means pure. My Nigerian name is Okeghene, which means gift of God. *Pure Gift of God.* I believe words have power, and names cause things to be. I couldn't help but wonder if naming me as she had was her way of trying to insulate me from my surroundings or cleanse them. Was purity what she wanted for herself? Was she afraid she might somehow taint me? And if I was a gift of God, was she a careless recipient who did not care for her gift well or was giving me up the greatest sacrifice she could have made?

My earliest memories of my mum were of her back as she was walking out the door. Leaving was familiar, well-rehearsed, and frequent. My mum left my father when I was a newborn. That's one time she left that I don't regret. She rescued me from a hostile environment. Who knows what unspeakable things might have happened to me—to both of us—if she had stayed.

If there is such a thing as luck, Mum didn't have any when it came to matters of the heart. She always wanted love, but it just never worked out. It was one tragic relationship after another, then another, like an addiction to heartbreak. But she still loved the idea of being in love.

We were both suckers for love stories, especially the movie *The Sound of Music*. We'd spend hours upon hours watching it together during my teens and early twenties. It was our favorite movie and one of the few things we could tolerate doing together for two hours and fifty-five minutes, including intermission. It was one of the few times we agreed on what love should look like, where our love met on common ground. We both loved the love story.

There was something about Maria that drew us both in, something familiar and painful. She was the mum I wanted, and the "woman adored" my mum wanted to be. As we sat watching, not talking, our hearts were both racing but for different reasons.

And then, of course, there was God, my mother's God. He was the One whose call creates conflict and makes you leave the ones you love or are supposed to love. Why does it have to be either-or? Maria knew my mother's God. He was the One calling her to become a nun, away from family and away from the hope of getting married and having children of her own. Maria doesn't see how she could fulfill her calling and be a wife and mother. So, she does what most people do when they are conflicted about their love for God. She ran away from the thing she felt was pulling her away from Him.

I remember watching as Maria returns to the womb-like confines of the convent. As she tells the Mother Abbess that she's ready to leave Captain von Trapp and the children behind and sacrifice her love for them on the altar of what she believes to be her calling, my stomach starts to churn. Something deep inside of me wants to scream, *No! You're making a mistake!* I involuntarily shoot a glance at my mother. She obviously enjoys this scene, and I resent her for it.

Have you ever been sitting in church and the preacher says something you always wanted to say but didn't have the nerve, and the person you want to say it to is right next to you? That's how I felt when Mother Abbess rejects Maria's decision to give herself exclusively to God. "These walls were not built to shut out problems. You have to face them. You have to live the life you were born to live."

I keep my head still, but I roll my eyes in my mother's direction. She's as oblivious to this tailor-made sermon as a sleeping child in church. Her decision was already made long ago. She sits glassy-eyed and hums along to the scene's closing song.

> Climb every mountain
> Ford every stream
> Follow every rainbow
> Till you find your dream

By the time Mother Abbess gets to the last lines of the song, my soul is shaking. I can't tell if it's hope or grief or fury I'm feeling.

> A dream that will need
> All the love you can give
> Every day of your life
> For as long as you live

Maria and I both listen to every word of the song. She finally gets what I've suspected ever since I was a small child. She realizes for the first time that the "dream that will need all the love you can give" is not God or what she believed to be her call to the convent. It is Georg Von Trapp and the children she adores. They are the ones who needed her the most. God did not need my mum. I did.

As many times as we watched this movie, we were seeing two very different love stories played out on the screen. My mother saw only the burgeoning love between a man and a woman. If she saw anything else, she didn't let on. For me it was the love of a mother towards her children, a love so strong, she would leave God within the cloistered walls of the church to be with the children she loved. My mother did just the opposite.

Sometimes I wonder if my mother struggled at all when she left me for God. I'd like to believe she did. It is possible that she faced the same internal conflict Maria did and felt she had to choose between God and family. And she chose God. Throughout her life, even before I was born and during my early years, she struggled with what she believed God wanted her to do. Choosing to leave me behind and serve God may have been what she saw as the lesser of two evils. In her mind, staying and ignoring what she believed to be the call of God would have been a much greater sin than leaving your only child.

Ignorance is the bliss of childhood. When my

mother left me with my grandparents, I was too young to have an opinion about it. She told everybody she was a missionary. I was too young to know what that meant. I'm still not sure what she meant by it.

My grandparents lived in Ozoro, about a three-hour drive from Benin City. It may as well have been another planet. Everything was so different. They believed in God, but their God was not so rigid and demanding. I was the first and only grandchild, so they really spoiled me, pampered me. At least that's what it felt like in contrast to how things were before.

I was four, old enough to know my mum left me, but young enough to believe it would not be for long. I lived with my grandparents in the main house, and there was a smaller house across the street. My grandmother had a lot of young people living there that she helped, and they would do odd chores around the place to help out. They were much older than me, but they would play with me. I was the apple of everybody's eyes.

My uncles and aunts would come and visit occasionally. I don't remember hearing from my mother or seeing her that much. Maybe she called and asked about me more times than I knew about, or maybe she talked to me once in a while. I don't really remember.

My grandmother worked at an all-girls secondary school teaching young girls how to cook and do all sorts of things. They would gather in a big kitchen-like room with silver ovens, and they would cluster at long tables covered in well-worn brightly colored vinyl. After some thorough instructions from my grandmother, they would cook or practice their baking, then wait with the nervous anticipation of novice chefs awaiting their first review. I was a welcome distraction to these "not quite women, not quite children." Some of them would hoist me on their hip and carry me around.

I still remember the smell of my grandmother's bread pudding. The warm spicy sweetness of the cinnamon and the buttery bread and raisin mixture would have me giddy with anticipation. She would make it for me often, and it was as if she would impart all of her affection for me into each delicious bite. It was a scrumptious delight that I love to this day because of my grandmother. I intentionally go to restaurants that have bread pudding on the dessert menu. Not a lot of places have it. I guess because it's more like an old-fashioned dessert.

"Karen, party of two? Your table is ready."

The sound rushed back into my ears, startling me like when you suddenly realize you were not paying attention to an ongoing conversation. I hadn't realized how lost in thought I was.

The Grand Lux was busy as usual. And as I

followed the hostess to the table, I exhaled, grateful that I didn't have to endure a long wait. I love this place. The lofty coffered ceilings and elegant décor are just upscale enough to make me feel like I'm giving myself a luxurious treat. I am getting better about taking care of myself, but I wasn't really much into any of that stuff in the earlier years.

Everything on the menu looked delicious, and my stomach growled in agreement. I looked it over out of courtesy or habit; I'm not sure which. I ordered promptly, already knowing what I wanted, and I was saving room for that. There was something soothing about the noisy ambience, the clinking of cutlery on plates. I relaxed into the plush velvet seating and waited for my meal to arrive. I found myself mesmerized by the deep mahogany of massive columns and the golden tones cast from the drum lighting. They were the colors of my family.

The server looked to be in her early twenties, just barely. For a quick minute, I remembered my days as a server, though it wasn't in any place as fancy as this.

"Salmon Three Ways? Careful, it's very, very hot."

I said a quick prayer and then practically inhaled the food. I felt a bit full, but I was determined to get what I came for. The server barely got a chance to finish asking if I wanted dessert.

"I'll have the warm sticky bun bread pudding, please."

"Oh, I'm sorry. It's not on the menu anymore."

It felt ridiculous for me to ask why. I mean, what difference would it make? This woman couldn't possibly know how much it meant to me. So, I feigned nonchalance.

"Oh. Okay. No problem."

Well, my temporary escape was over. There was nothing left to do but head home. But I just couldn't shake the feeling of disappointment. It reminded me of a line I heard from a movie recently, "Life gets easier if you don't want so much." I was well trained in disappointment. The few times my mum visited me during my years at my grandmother's house, I would think, "Oh, mummy's come for me!" only to realize that was not the case. Once again, I'd see her back going through the door without me.

Disappointment only comes to those who have expectations of others who are either incapable of meeting them or unwilling. The reality is, sometimes it's not that our expectations are so high that the person who disappointed us misses, but it's that the person's expectation of themselves is so low they hit it every time. And we don't have the power to control anyone's expectations of themselves.

None of us gets it right all the time, parents included. The most we can do is to expect the best. That doesn't make us immune to disappointment when they don't live up to our expectations. But as adults, it does afford us the privilege of approaching every situation like it's a fresh start. If not for them, for you. That's the unselfish side of love that I'm not entirely comfortable with yet.

Selfishness is something we inherit and pass on to our children. Every single one of us is born selfish. It's an innate survival instinct. We're born making demands, especially of our mothers, and we carry that sense of entitlement throughout life. Fathers are supposed to be there, but we'll figure out a way to get by if they're not. We'll make excuses for them to make their absence a little more tolerable. *He was a drunk; he was no good; he wasn't ready to be a father.* But with mothers, we are much less forgiving. They brought us into this world. And it just seems like there's some unwritten law somewhere that says they're supposed to help us get through it. We expect her selfishness to end when ours begins.

2

BIRDS OF FLIGHT

Outside, I heard the gurgled scream of what I thought was a man. My young mind had not yet learned how to identify the sounds of such violence, and for a moment, it threw me into a daze. We were all in a one-room bungalow, a square thing with three big windows on the back wall. My aunt with the baby, my three other cousins, the helper, and I all moved at once like a flock of birds, each to one of the windows.

There on the ground was a man writhing like a snake. His back was arched, trying in vain to escape the next blow. Soldiers in camouflage stood by watching, anxious to get their turn. The soldier in the coveted position stood over the man, a barbed wire whip in one hand, a rifle dangling in the other. I inhaled sharply at the sound of the whip whistling through the air then slashing across the man's body. I was sure the worst thing imaginable was happening to him, this unbearable torment from which there was no escape.

With each scream, it was as if every breath in his body gathered to force out the sound of his pain, hoping somebody would hear it and help him. I heard it, but there was nothing I could do but watch. I didn't want to, but my feet were riveted to the spot, and the sound of his pain begged me not to look away. So, I just stood there and watched him being tortured. This was our new life.

The military prison camp was surrounded by high walls with rolls of barbed wire on top. The place where they had tortured the man was grassy and open, just like a football field. It was an almost obscene sight, that patch of green surrounded by all the steel gray and concrete. The community we were in was large, and there were other houses, but we really didn't talk to anyone or interact. It was just us and that bungalow, a prison within a prison.

We were allowed to go to school. In the beginning, soldiers would escort us there and back. But after a while they figured we weren't going anywhere, so they let us go and come on our own. But not my aunt. She couldn't go anywhere at all. It was hard to believe that just three years earlier, I was entering into one of the happiest times of my life.

I was seven years old when I was taken to Lagos to live with my aunt and uncle, my mum's younger brother. They lived about twenty-four hours away from my grandparents' house in Ozoro, the place I had come to know as my home. My grandparents were getting older, and with my grandfather's health declining, they thought it would be best for me to be with younger parents. Mum was still in America, living a life alien to my own.

The hustle and bustle of Lagos filled me with wonder. It was a fast-paced and vibrant city humming with activity. I had never seen so many people in one place. My uncle and aunt had three kids, all younger than me. After I moved in, eventually, they had another baby. I loved being an instant big sister. Living with my uncle and aunt, I had my first glimpse of what a loving parent-child relationship looked like. I was treated no differently than their own biological children, and my cousins were more like my brothers and sisters. They were my family.

While I lived with my aunt and uncle, mum would visit every now and again. I'd gotten used to her absence being the dominant presence in my life, but I was always happy to see her. At times I would think she would be taking me back with her to wherever she was going. As happy as I was with my aunt and uncle, it would still hurt when I realized she was leaving without me. The only thing that made the pain bearable was being with my extended family. Life with them was sweet, that is until that dreadful day when everything changed.

My uncle was in the army and had gotten involved in an unsuccessful military coup. He was a marked man, so he ended up having to flee the country. None of us knew about the coup, not even my aunt. He didn't tell us. He just did it secretly with some of his friends. Thankfully, he was able to escape, but we were not so fortunate.

The soldiers came in broad daylight. The rumble of their military trucks marked the end of the world as we knew it, and they rounded us up like cattle and placed us under arrest. We weren't allowed to take anything with us, just the clothes on our backs and a few supplies for the baby. There were no explanations offered, just a long bumpy ride in the back of the truck and lots of tears.

Life was miserable on the military base, especially for my aunt. As kids, we adjusted and coped as best as we could. We would play with each other and dance and sing songs. We at least had some freedom to move about and go to school and the market. But my aunt was under heavy surveillance, and she wasn't allowed to go anywhere at all.

Our helper's name was Alice, like Alice in Wonderland. She had been with the family for many years, and even though she was given a choice to leave, she chose to be locked up with us over her own freedom. So, all seven of us lived in that one-room bungalow. Life took on a new normal, and as one day blurred into the next, before we knew it, an entire year had passed. Then one day, as abruptly as we had been snatched away from our home, we were removed from the base and taken to a new location.

They moved us to another small one-story bungalow, and the armed soldiers from the military base were replaced by police officers armed with guns. My aunt still was not allowed to go anywhere, but we could go to school, and Alice was allowed to go to the market. The police guards were lazy, and after seeing us every day for a year, they got too comfortable. Sometimes they would leave early or not show up at all. Little did they know, we were carefully planning our escape, and their carelessness would give us the perfect opportunity.

My uncle had settled safely in America. Physically, we were oceans apart, but we never left his thoughts, and he was determined to get us out of there. We had a friend, a beautiful Indian girl who owned a Chinese restaurant. We called her Anju, and she lived on top of the restaurant. She was the link that my uncle used to communicate with us, and I became the carrier pigeon.

On a day just like any other day, I took the twenty-minute walk from school to Anju's restaurant. It had become a familiar route, and I welcomed the break from the monotony of life under house arrest. There were no visible signs of imprisonment on me, but caution was my constant companion, and for me, it was as tangible as manacles on my feet. I was still a prisoner.

As I entered the restaurant, the cool air greeted me at the door, and for a moment I lost myself in the aroma of sesame oil, garlic, ginger, and seared meat. Anju spotted me at the entrance and smiled as I made my way to an inconspicuous spot to wait.

The atmosphere was a peculiar and wonderful fusion of cultures. Anju's thick Indian accent floating through the crowd, tables peppered with brightly colored dishes, and the random chatter of a melting pot of people enjoying or waiting to enjoy their food.

At the first opportunity, Anju made her way to where I was. After we greeted each other, she took my notebook and wrote the message my uncle had given her from an earlier phone call. I wasn't really interested in what she was writing. I was too busy taking everything else in and wishing I could stay a little longer. She handed the notebook back to me and gave me a long hug.

"Be careful."

She smelled warm and spicy, like the restaurant. I smiled and nodded, then weaved my way around the tables toward the door. Just before I stepped into the bright afternoon sunlight, I glanced over my shoulder. I'm not sure why I did it. Maybe subconsciously I felt Anju's eyes still on me. She was standing where I'd left her, arms akimbo, and she made a slight motion with her head as if gently nudging me through the door.

As soon as I got back to the bungalow, I handed the notebook over to my aunt. She tore out the page with the message and took a few steps over to the other side of the room to read it by herself. I never knew what my aunt did with those messages, if she read and then destroyed them. But piece by piece, on pages of ripped out notebook paper, my uncle's elaborate plan was put into place.

On the day of our escape, the guards had left early. We went to bed at our usual time, me on a mattress on the floor with Alice and my three oldest cousins, and my aunt on the big bed with the baby. Nothing appeared out of the ordinary, except we all had our regular clothes on. Late in the middle of the night, my aunt woke us up. Without a word, we knew it was time to go.

There was a water pump behind the bungalow, so we often went back there to fetch water. There was also a back road there that led to the main road. With nothing but the clothes we were wearing, we slipped out the back and started the fifteen-minute walk to the market-place. We moved as silent as the night and doubled our steps to keep up with my aunt. The baby was swaddled snugly on her back, and the Fulani head-dress she wore to hide her face and hair flowed from her brisk movement.

My heart outran my footsteps as we approached the taxi stand. It was busy, but not like the middle of the day. After a brief exchange between my aunt and one of the drivers, we crowded into his cab. It would be nearly three hours before we crossed the border into the Republic of Benin. My stomach tightened as the car creaked and swayed. There was nothing to see or do except listen to the rumbling of the tires on the road, which eventually lulled me into a deep sleep.

The following morning, the guards arrived at the bungalow as usual. Alice busied herself with chores throughout the day and left the tv on so no one would suspect anything. As soon as the guards left for the day, she used the same back road we had used the night before and escaped to her hometown. By the time anyone suspected anything, we would all be long gone.

When we arrived in Benin, my uncle had arranged for us to stay at a little hotel and sent a man to come and help us. He had passports for all of us. This was back in the days when it was relatively easy to get a visa, and within three days, we were boarding a plane to America.

The man stayed with us the whole time and led us so we would know what to do. He was on the same plane with us, but we acted like we didn't know him, and he kept his distance just in case we got caught.

It's amazing how our lives can be so drastically altered because of decisions we never made or were privy to. Here I was barely twelve years old, and I had already spent three years imprisoned, eight years separated from my biological mother, and was now a virtual asylum seeker. I saw things I never wanted to see, heard things I never wanted to hear, experienced things I'd just as soon forget. And the hardest part is, I had absolutely no say in the matter.

These were hard lessons to learn at such a young age—at any age—and even harder to unlearn as I got older. This must be what some people call generational curses, decisions that are made that predispose you to trauma and cycles that you have to be intentional about disrupting. Unfortunately, bad memories stick better than good. There are memories that we revisit and others that we lay to rest. Like a sieve, we have to sift the past and make sure only the best of it remains.

As the plane made its ascent, I could feel the fear of getting caught draining out of me, diminishing as quickly as the dotted landscape beneath us until we were safely out of reach. And just like that, I flew away from the torture field, our years of imprisonment, and into the life of a mother I barely knew.

3

THE CURSE OF ALONENESS

The open casket was couched between two large sprays of gladioli, roses, and chrysanthemums. The shock of the white floral arrangements against the dimly lit backdrop cast a heavenly glow across the front of the sanctuary. Interspersed between the flowers were large portraits capturing the different seasons of the woman whose life the crowds had come to celebrate.

One by one, thousands of mourners young and old streamed past to pay their respects, some lingering to take one last look. After the casket was closed and shrouded in fragrant bouquets, select clergy, friends, and family members were called to share reflections of her life. They spoke of a life well-lived, a devoted wife, an exemplary leader, a skilled administrator. But there was one common thread in every tribute: Lois Irene Evans had made family a priority.

The memorial service was over four hours long and filled with nothing but glowing words about the wonderful wife and mother she had been and how special she made them all feel. She had four children, thirteen grandchildren, and three great-grandchildren, and all who spoke agreed that she had made a profound and lasting impact on their lives.

My mind traveled back over the last twenty-eight years, stopping at all the emotional landmarks I had erected in my heart. As I continued watching the live stream of the televised service, the laudations continued, and I could feel the pulse of anger throbbing in the veins of my neck. With all this woman had accomplished and had been involved in, she still managed to be there for her kids. What was my mother's excuse?

It was the summer of 1992 when we arrived in New York. We shuffled down the airless tunnel-like corridor beyond the glass panel walls and made our way to customs. The uneasy feeling in my stomach returned as we approached the customs officer. We all did our best to look as natural as possible, as if we had made this trip a hundred times before. To my surprise, we breezed through the brief interview and were granted access to a whole new world.

"Enjoy your stay!"

I was too nervous to return the smile of the officer. My thoughts were already drifting towards the long-awaited reunion.

My uncle was already waiting for us in the baggage claim area, and there beside him stood my mother. As we approached, I avoided eye contact with her and focused instead on my uncle's familiar face. He swallowed us in hugs and teary-eyed grins as, one by one, he welcomed us into our new homeland. Then it was my mother's turn. She pulled me close as if reclaiming ownership of something precious she had lost. I was happy to see her, but I couldn't help but stiffen slightly as she wrapped her arms around me.

We lingered as long as we could, but my uncle, aunt and cousins had to make their connecting flight. I had been separated from my uncle for the past two years, and now after five years of living with my aunt and cousins as my closest family, I was about to be separated from them for the first time. We clung to each other and squeezed out our goodbyes and promises to see each other soon. As they headed towards the terminal, I swallowed hard and followed my mother out the automatic doors.

My new home was in Staten Island, about a forty-minute drive from the airport. Mum gripped the steering wheel, and at first, she made small talk as if she were trying to catch up for the last eight years.

"You're going to love it here!"

She kept her eyes straight ahead and I suspect she was trying to convince herself more than me. I curled my mouth into a half-smile and stared out the window. The sound of the radio made the silence that was now between us even more awkward. I was a jumble of emotions. I missed my cousins and aunt so much that it made my stomach hurt, and I wasn't sure what to expect of my new home. Would it be perfectly manicured lawns and houses with white picket fences like in the magazines? My imagination ran wild, but as we passed through and out of the areas that bear any faint resemblance to anything you might see on the glossy pages of a magazine, my daydreams vanished into thin exhaust-polluted air.

The area had an oppressed mood. I later discovered it was a hub for mafia activity. Mum lived in a portion of an old house that had been converted into a small two-bedroom apartment, not much bigger than the prison bungalows where I'd lived for the past two years. As we entered the small living room, a noisy box fan rattled away in the apartment's only window. I looked through the grid of the fan onto the car lined street and wondered what my cousins were doing. It had been a long and exhausting day, and I was relieved when my mother showed me to the room that I would call my own. As I lay in bed, staring through the darkness at my new surroundings, across the hall I heard the soft click of the door to the room that my mother shared with husband #3.

He was a man she knew from Nigeria who had told her, "God said you're my wife," and she believed it. Once again, this God of hers was speaking in a confused language I didn't understand. This one was a marriage of convenience. She thought she would get a husband, and he thought he would get a way to change his immigration status. Only one of them was right. After she brought him to America, they started a small church together. But she soon realized he was nothing more than a slick-talking womanizer, and she found herself in the same abusive cycle of domestic violence that she was in with her first two husbands.

There was no time to adjust to my new environment. I landed right in the middle of daily drama. I had waited eight years to be reunited only to discover I was living with a sad and deeply depressed woman who was married to a man who never wanted her in the first place. Physically she was present, but emotionally, she was only available to God. Prayer was her drug of choice, her only escape from the reality of the loveless world she lived in. Husband #3 stayed long enough to get what he wanted and then left for the arms of another woman. My presence was eclipsed by my mother's own dissatisfied life, and I was left to fend for myself in a new country, a new home, and an environment that was hostile to anything foreign.

Life with my mother was as unstable as water. She called it "living by faith," which translated to never having any money and a whole lot of stress. I quickly learned not to take things for granted like having electricity or being able to get back into the apartment after school. The lights got turned off regularly because bills were rarely paid on time. And I got so used to coming home from school to find the locks changed that, after a while, I didn't even react. I just sat on the front steps and waited. Mum spent her time devoted to prayer and trying to keep the church she and her ex-husband started afloat. She threw herself into ministry and pastoring full time, so concerned about the souls of others that she couldn't see the troubled soul that was right in front of her. Prayer and God's work took first and second place in her life. She would drop everything for that, including me.

We bounced around from one place to another, her dodging landlords and unpaid rent and me changing schools. Finally, we ended up in Harlem, a concrete jungle of old houses all sandwiched together and corner stores and store-front churches littering the streets. Leaving the mafia-influenced streets of Staten Island behind was a slightly happier prospect. Still, the thought of transferring to a school in Harlem and being treated like an outsider all over again was unbearable. I chose instead to make the ninety-minute commute by train and ferry to Staten Island and back each day.

My mother never showed any interest in my school work or anything I was doing. I transitioned into my teen years with no real guidance and her barely noticing. When I saw a man lying in a pool of blood, a victim of a drive-by mafia hit in my old neighborhood, she wasn't emotionally available to provide any comfort. I couldn't tell her about the kids who made fun of me because of my accent or who bullied me because I couldn't afford to get new school clothes. I couldn't share with her how ugly and insecure I felt or talk to her about how I was always trying to fit in and be like other people. We were both lonely and abandoned in each other's company.

I didn't want to be tough, but I had no other choice. I knew that if I needed anything, physical or emotional, I was on my own. I started working at McDonald's when I was fourteen. It only paid $50 a month, but that was enough to pay for school supplies and other personal items I needed. When the paychecks started coming, I discovered the one way my mother was sure to always give me her attention, when she needed money.

Money became the connection between my mother and me. She leaned on me for both emotional and financial support as though I were some strange aberration of a surrogate husband. I went from instant big sister with my cousins, which I loved, to instant provider, first for myself and then for both of us. Teenage years were difficult enough without the added pressure of carrying such a heavy burden.

Mum always had money trouble. Either she didn't have any, or "by faith," she spent what she didn't have and ended up with debts that I had to bail her out of. As I got older, and later all through college, I started working two or three jobs at a time so I could help her. The more independent I became, the more dependent she was on me to pay all of her bills. It always felt like I was the mother and she was the child.

By the time my mother shifted her attention to me, I was well into my twenties, and by then, I didn't feel like I needed it anymore. I was already living in the well-worn groove of making it on my own, hustling to take care of myself, paying her bills, or bailing her out of whatever new dilemma she had gotten herself into. Except for one time she didn't want me to bail her out.

Mum was a businesswoman, and she had developed

a certain set of skills when it came to paying those she was doing business with. Some might call it negotiating, but it was more like masterful manipulation. She would bargain for the agreement, but when it came time to pay, she would say, "Oh, that's not what we agreed on." There were times she would conveniently abandon a business to get back to her work for God, usually leaving a trail of debt behind. She always owed people money, and somebody or another was always taking her to court for some unpaid debt. On this particular occasion, it was a company with which she had done business. They had done some work for her and she didn't have the money to pay them, so they took her to court and won. Later, on the day of the court hearing, my phone rang.

"I'm going to be in jail for the next few days, but don't tell anybody." Click.

It was a couple of days before Christmas. What was I supposed to tell her brothers when they phoned? Mum was tough when she wanted to be, or maybe it was stubbornness. Either way, she made up her mind that she would rather spend three days in a lonely prison cell than pay up. She didn't give me a chance to bail her out. This time, she didn't want me to. The only thing she wanted was for me to preserve her pride and not let anybody know about it. That was how I spent Christmas that year, in my apartment worrying about how she was doing in jail and nervous about covering up her secret. That's the way it always was. Me and her going through crazy stuff that no one else knew about.

My mother was "living by faith." Maybe that's what gave her courage knowing that she was taking her faith and her God into the cell with her. She had faith I didn't understand. Her faith left us deprived, dirt poor, and in a constant state of threatened repossession or litigation. Her faith got the lights turned off and got us kicked from place to place because she couldn't keep up with the rent. Her faith kept her wrapped up in prayer to the neglect of everything else. I didn't know or understand this faith. All I knew was that I didn't want to be like the flaws I saw in her.

Lois Evans was only two years older than my mother. As I watched the conclusion of the memorial service, I couldn't help but wish my mother had been more like her. True enough, Lois had a great husband, money, and maybe less trauma in her background, but it was obvious that motherhood was one responsibility and privilege this woman was passionate about. Mum had only one child and a tiny ministry, yet I never ranked high enough on her priority list for her to take care of me at the most critical times in my life.

Most parents do everything they can to help their

children and see to it that they have what they need both physically and emotionally. They see their children as gifts, and caring for them until they release them into the world a privilege. But it was never that way with my mother. Yes, she saw me as a gift, but I was a gift that she re-purposed for herself. She gave birth to me, but from the start, she believed that I was there to help her. In her mind, that's what I was put on earth for. So, when I went to live with her, I became the answer to everything she was lacking. She was supposed to have the answers to my questions, or at least be able to tell me where to find them. She was supposed to take care of me, not me always taking care of her. I was supposed to be able to lean on her, but it was always her leaning on me and me leaning on whatever I could find to keep from toppling over.

Our mother-daughter trust was broken from the start. Trust is like glass. Once it's broken, even if you can somehow glue it back together, the cracks are still visible. I thought that when I went to live with my mother she would fill in all the cracks for me and that life with her would bear some semblance of normalcy. Instead, my relationship with her was like a fourth marriage: toxic, dysfunctional, and damaged. She was no Lois Evans. There's really no point in comparing her to anyone else because no matter what other mothers' accomplishments are, they're not my mother; she is. I just had to play with the cards I was dealt.

One day, I took a long hard look at her, and I realized that this is as good as it's going to get. I didn't want to sugarcoat the truth because when you sugarcoat the truth, your heart gets cavities. I had to face the fact that she was never going to be the ideal mother. She's never going to be there for me. She's always going to be dependent on me and believe that's the way it's supposed to be. I stopped waiting for her to pay a debt that she just didn't have the emotional currency to pay.

Some mothers understand what it means to be a mother; others are mothers by default. The biological connection will always be there, but like an umbilical cord, only the stump of a relationship remains. I could live my life demanding in one way or another that my mother become what she was not, or I could make up my mind to become everything I once needed her to be. I understand that there's a why behind every what. There's a reason she acted and thought the way she did, though I may never know what those reasons were. But what I do know is that sometimes the best you comes out of knowing who you don't want to become.

4

THE DAY I MET GOD

L ife is a series of endings and beginnings. From the moment we're born, we start to leave our mothers. It's what's supposed to happen. There is a severing that must take place, an ending of one relationship so that another phase of that relationship can begin. The health of the relationship depends on it. When that separation does not happen, something hardens, and the connection gets infected, like an umbilical cord that doesn't drop off.

I was my mother's right arm, and it had been that way for so long that it was hard for me to imagine it being any different. I was well into my twenties, and we were now living in the Bronx. There was never anything stated, just this knowing that I was expected to always be there for her. I had my own car, my own money, but it was as though I was tethered with just enough length to get to college and back. Just as I thought I was old enough and grown enough to strike out on my own, another crisis would arise and snatch me back to my mother's side.

Guilt is a difficult addiction to break. I would fool myself into believing that I could leave at any time, but then I would think, how's she going to pay her bills? And I would push the key into the lock and find myself on the wrong side of independence once again. There was never really much for me to look forward to. When I wasn't working or studying, I was with my mother at some prayer meeting or another. Occasionally I would date, but I was never really interested in any of the guys. There was never any real connection.

In the meantime, my twenties were running away from me, and my dream of getting married and having a bunch of kids was starting to feel as elusive as my freedom. My mother was perfectly okay with me giving up my life for hers. She felt justified in her dependence on me. In her mind, that's why I was born, to help her. It never occurred to her that she was supposed to encourage me to go and live my own life. She clipped my wings with the scissors of emotional blackmail and my sense of duty as a daughter. I would have remained there like a caged bird if it hadn't been for the incident that my mother later described as ruining our relationship.

My mother's mother came to visit us in New York. She had always been a very direct, straight to the point kind of person, and this time was no exception. We were in the living room, and without warning or any preliminary conversation, she delivered her own emancipation proclamation.

"You know, you've got to go live your life. You've got to get away from your mother and go get married."

She locked her gaze on my face as if by some divine impartation she was transferring courage into me. I stood there dumbfounded. I could hardly believe what I had just heard. Was this really my mother's mother telling me to get away from her own daughter? My grandmother had assessed the situation between my mother and me and had seen enough to know that this was not a mutually beneficial arrangement. Just like that, with those two simple statements, she validated my right to have a life of my own. She unlocked my guilt cage, and I jumped on the first opportunity to go to Houston to get my Ph.D. But little did I know that before I left, I would have an appointment with God.

There was nothing unusual about me going with my mother to every prayer meeting. Sometimes she would pray all through the night, and I'd be right there with her. After so many years of accompanying her and listening to her prayers, I learned to pray too. At first it was more by rote, me mimicking what I had seen and heard her do so many times. But somewhere along the way, my prayers took on meaning. My mum's passion for prayer started to rub off on me, and I started to understand to a small degree this attraction to talking to God that she had. Prayer became like therapy for me. It was an opportunity for me to talk about things I wouldn't normally talk about, things that felt too big for me to handle on my own. It felt safe because He never talked back until the night my one-way conversation came to an end.

There was one prayer request that always stayed on my heart. "God, am I ever going to find somebody to love?" One particular night, I was at a prayer meeting with my mother as usual, and one of the pastors came over to pray for me. All of a sudden, he stopped praying to God about me and started talking to me directly.

"A year from now, you will meet your husband. He is somebody you already know."

I could feel the hair standing on the back of my neck. It was as though he had eavesdropped on my prayer request, because there he was talking to me about a conversation only God and I knew about. He was a pastor, yes, but this was just a regular guy, not anybody I would have thought would be God's personal spokesperson.

I started doing a quick mental review of all the guys I knew. I wasn't sure who he meant because everyone I'd ever dated was a jerk, and I didn't want any of them. But there was something about the certainty and finality of what he said that gave me hope. I grabbed onto that message and held on like it was the last life preserver on a sinking ship. This, for me, was novel information. The God who took my mother away from me, who stole all the attention she should have given to me and left me bereft of love, was now promising me someone of my very own to love. However ironic and incredible it seemed, I believed it.

I became like a woman obsessed. I decided I would not date anyone. I would just wait for this man I was supposed to meet in a year. My family couldn't understand how I was going to meet somebody if I wasn't dating, but my mind was made up. I figured I might as well start preparing for the wedding, so I started ordering wedding stuff and requesting information from wedding vendors. When they would ask, "what's your groom's name?" I would say, "God's Best." I didn't know what else to call him because I had no idea who he was. I'm sure they must have thought I was crazy.

I left for Houston to pursue my Ph.D. with my grandmother's words still ringing in my ears. It was as though she gave me permission to leave. For the first time in my adult life, I felt like things were starting to look up for me. I was finally on my own, by my own choice this time, and the prospect of love was on the horizon. I had no idea it would come to me in white socks.

When I was a young girl back in Nigeria, when I still lived with my aunt and uncle, there was a teacher I loved. She had five boys, and I got to know one of them because he was in the same class as me. I wasn't interested in him or anything like that, but I loved how white his socks were. I would marvel at how his mom always kept them so clean. They were super white, like a Hollywood smile. I couldn't help but notice.

Some time after I had settled down in Houston, I received a Facebook message from none other than "white socks." We hadn't seen or heard from each other in over fifteen years since I left Africa. I was surprised he remembered me because he was nowhere on my radar. I didn't even remember his name until I saw it in my inbox. He was in Dallas pursuing his master's degree, and I was the first person he searched for after arriving in America. He had been thinking about me all this time. It was exactly a year after the pastor had prayed for me. Three months later, we were married.

Leaving my mother was the best decision I ever made, but it wasn't an easy one. I felt like I was abandoning her to get married and have a life of my own. I had never even thought of leaving my mother until my grandmother said it. But thanks to her, I recognized the need to put distance between myself and an unhealthy relationship. The struggle was between my guilt in leaving her and my entitlement to a life without my mother always being the number one priority. I realized it was a necessity. I had to outgrow one relationship to grow into another. I needed to prioritize my life and stop taking responsibility for the life she wanted but never had. The umbilical cord had to be cut.

Happiness is a choice, and I couldn't make that choice for my mother. That was something only she could do for herself. After all, it is not the responsibility of the child to make the parent happy. It is not my responsibility to fill any void in her life or to fulfill her needs. That's a God-sized vacancy that only He can fill. The sooner I realized that, the better and more meaningful my life became. It would have been unfair to her for me to continue to enable her dependency. I had to go.

The hardest line to draw is a boundary line, especially when the other person believes they have a right to cross it. Boundaries say this far and no more. Without them, your life becomes like a house with no deed and no locks. Anyone can come in and possess it. That's what my mother did. I don't think she meant to completely take over my life. She just didn't know where else to go.

Leaving my mother was the ultimate 'no.' It was the only way I could say 'yes' to me, and in a strange way, to a newfound relationship with God. He wasn't just my mother's God anymore. I no longer saw Him as someone who was just observing me in my misery. If I had established healthy boundaries sooner, I could have avoided some of the turmoil I experienced. Looking back, I can see how God was working out some of the details of my life, despite my lack of boundaries, using the broken pieces to lead me to a better life.

When a child is born, the umbilical cord is cut. No one asks the child or the mother if that's what they want. In a similar way, it seemed the tables were turned. In the beginning, God took my mother away from me. Then, when I was finally ready to fly, He took me away from my mother. I am not suggesting that it is okay to remain in a miserable situation and wait for God to do something when you have the power to do something about it. It is our parents' obligation to prepare us for adulthood. It is our responsibility to embrace adulthood with or without their support.

Mum once told me that God sent me to help her and that she may be of help to me one day. I had no idea what she meant, especially since I was always the one helping her. All this time, I thought God was my enemy, monopolizing my mother's time in prayer. But maybe some of those prayers had been for me, and they were working after all.

5

FACING MORTALITY

"Karen. Karen."

I squeezed my eyes shut a little longer. It felt like I had only just fallen into a good sleep after several interruptions earlier that night. I took a deep breath, let it out with a sigh, and hated my eyes for opening before I felt ready. The numbers on the digital clock glared at me. It was 3:41 in the morning. I sighed again and shifted my legs out from under the warm covers, careful not to wake my husband.

"Karen?"

I could hear the confusion and panic rising in her voice. She sounded like a little girl lost in a crowd of strangers. The hallway was dark, but I knew my way. I'd done this so many times before.

"Ma? What's wrong?"

She was standing in the middle of the room. For a moment, I wasn't sure if she had been on her way to try to leave the room or was about to get back into the bed. As I got closer, I could see the reason she was up. I sat her down in the chair and started pulling the sheets off the bed, piling them on the floor. She looked so small sitting there, so helpless.

My thoughts drifted back to the conversation we had a few days earlier.

"I couldn't cope with being a mother."

We were on the way to her doctor's appointment. Mum had lost sight in one eye and was quickly losing sight in the other. This was unlike our usual conversations. It was peaceful. For the first time in my forty years of living, we were communicating.

"I know I've always been some source of trouble for you."

I could hardly believe what I was hearing. For a moment, I had the same feeling I did years before when I was leaving the airport with her, like I was venturing into brand new territory. This was the first time my mom had ever come this close to an apology or admitted how difficult life with her had been for me.

My mother never took care of her health throughout her life. She managed to avoid visits to the doctor's office by standing firm on her conviction that Jesus was the only doctor she needed. It was only a matter of time before age and neglect caught up to her. And when it did, it stormed into her life in the form of a stroke that left her incapacitated and unable to live on her own.

It had taken me years to pluck up enough courage to leave my mother, and I needed help to do that. The thought of living with her again went through me like an icy chill, but the doctor had made it clear that she could not live by herself. The thought of putting her in a nursing home never crossed my mind. I had no choice but to move her into our new house with us. However, I was not expecting her to bring housemates along.

When mum moved in, she brought two uninvited guests with her. The first was a massive seizure that showed up two months after she moved in. By the time she left the hospital, the second guest was accompanying her. Mum had been diagnosed with dementia. She had always been very stubborn, but dementia took her obstinance to a whole new level. Initially, everything was a fight. She refused her insulin. She rejected her wheelchair. She argued and complained incessantly. She was drowning in a sea of forgetfulness and clutching at the remnants of her independence the only way she knew how.

You can't reason with dementia. It swings like a

pendulum from one end of the emotional spectrum to the other. You're never really sure which extreme will show up or if it will land somewhere in between. It's moody and hostile one moment, cheerful or frightened by the slightest movement the next. It plays with lucidity like a game of peek-a-boo, giving you glimpses of a stranger you hate being around, or the person you once knew, or the person you wished her to be. At times it's like dealing with a spoiled child that always wants to have its own way. At other times, it's like a woman whose hormones have gone on a rampage, angry and irrational one minute, depressed and melancholic the next. Sometimes everything goes quiet and vacant as if a squatter has taken possession of the mind and put up a fence to keep everyone out, including the owner. Then there are those all too frequent moments when it's like having a helpless baby for whom you have to do every-thing and who demands all of your attention.

Dementia is merciless. It demands all of your time. It has no regard for anyone, not even its host. It doesn't care how tired or stressed you are. It doesn't matter if you've run up and down the stairs twenty-five times only to be asked each time why the room is different. It transforms televisions into monsters and imprisons you in a room where you can't recognize the door. It can give you a week of relative normalcy, then just as you feel like you're catching your breath, you get a follow-up week or two filled with enough meanness to make up for the week that was missed. It forces you to get dressed, impressing a sense of urgency in getting somewhere, then it snatches the destination and leaves you clueless as to what you were just doing.

It's heart-wrenching to watch someone you love succumb to the tireless grip of dementia, to see them come to terms with being absent against their will. Mum had no choice but to deal with the reality that she had to relinquish her freedom, her adulthood, her life as she knew it, and yet still keep living. Part of me blamed her for the suffering she was experiencing. But even if I felt like she should have taken better care of herself, it wouldn't change anything.

"I couldn't cope with being a mother." Now I was beginning to understand what she meant, or at least my interpretation of it. In earlier years, there were times I took my mother's absence personally, thinking I somehow had something to do with her leaving me behind. But it really wasn't about me. It was about her perception of herself. I believe that my presence compelled her to look into a mirror that reflected every-thing she felt she was not. From my vantage point, moth-erhood was like dementia for her, an undeniable reality that made her feel lost, deficient, and out of control.

Dementia only amplified what I had experienced most of my life, that I had expectations of my mum that she was incapable of fulfilling. I expected her to take care of me growing up and to make my needs a priority. I expected or at least wanted her to understand that now that I have two small children, a husband, and a demanding job, I could not possibly give her all my time.

Dementia forced me to finally put my expectations of my mother to rest, and in general, to release my expectations of people I have no power to change. God in His sovereignty has limited and focused my power to change only myself and those over whom I have authority, specifically my children. And that's only for a time. The fact that my mother did not exercise her privilege to be an intentional and positive change agent in my life while she could is no longer of any consequence. Where her power ended, mine began. It's up to me now to learn from her mistakes. Watching my mum decline in health motivated me to take better care of my own. Her imperfections and shortcomings as a mother have made me determined to be the best mother that I can be to my two little girls. Perfection is not the goal. Improvement is.

Improvement is one of the few things that requires us to consider our past. The difference between improvement and resentment is the intention. If my only reason for looking at the way things were is to rehearse the pain, that only serves as fertilizer for roots of bitterness in my life. But if I look at where I've been and what I've experienced in life to see what changes I can make to improve myself, then my past becomes the catalyst for my progress. Nothing in my past can keep me down or hold me back anymore, because I realize that I am my most powerful change agent, not my mother.

Life is a series of "next things." Like walking, you can only take one step at a time. No matter how much you try to see what's ahead, how near or how far, you can only take one step at a time. Dementia is a marathon, and marathoners don't focus on the finish line. They focus on the mile they're in. This has been an invaluable truth in managing the demands of dementia. If I think beyond the next step, I feel overwhelmed, stressed, and discouraged. But the next step is manageable.

I glanced at the clock next to mum's bed. It was 4:13 a.m. Everything was clean and dry. Mum was already dozing, probably tuckered out by the quick wash-up and change of clothes. I stood there for a moment just looking at her. I felt no anger, no resentment, just a calm resolve. I had made it through the next thing. The only thing left to do was to get her back in bed.

I got close and spoke in softened tones so as not to startle her.

"Okay, Ma."

As she roused, I slipped my arm behind her to get a firm enough hold to ease her out of the chair, and we staggered over to the bed. As I lowered her against the pillow and drew the covers up, the words of a song I'd heard earlier came floating up to my mind.

> Sometimes discouraged, but not
> defeated,
> Cast down, but not destroyed,
> There are times I don't understand
> But I believe it's turning around for me.
> I've had struggles and disappointments
> There are times I felt so alone
> Some of my friends, they let me down
> But I still believe it's turning around
> for me.

As I made the walk back down the dark hallway to my room, I cringed at the thought of having to get back up in less than two hours. I was exhausted, but more than anything, I felt an overwhelming sense of gratitude that I could find my way down a dark hallway to my intended destination, independent and unsupported. As I slipped in between the sheets, the final refrain of the song became my hopeful prayer.

And it won't always be like this;
He will perfect that concerning me.
And sooner or later it will turn in my
    favor;
It's turning around for me.

6

RESTING IN PEACE

The gymnasium was buzzing with excitement and the murmurs of many nations. A third of the rafters were filled to capacity as the M.O. Campbell Education Center in Houston was transformed into a virtual Ellis Island. More than two thousand immigrants had gathered for this long-awaited day, the day they would finally become American citizens. Some, already brimming with anticipated patriotism, were carrying miniature U.S. flags. Others were contemplative as if reminiscing on their own unique story of the journey that would both end and begin in this place. Among the candidates sat my mother with me accompanying her.

The wait had been long, nearly three hours, plenty of time to sit and visit with old memories. Mum talked about how troubled her entire life had been, her battle with depression, and the abuse she experienced in her marriages. Then, as if working in reverse, the subject of my childhood surfaced. Whenever we broached this subject, mum would get defensive. It had always seemed as though she wanted to convince her heart that she had been the best mother, but her mind would object. The conflict this created would usually manifest in some form of tangible tension. She never liked any kind of criticism or anything that reminded her that she did less than a perfect job. I suppose that's true for all of us. No one wants to be reminded of their failures. The present always places us beyond the threshold of changing the past.

The judge sat, hands folded, behind a skirted table draped in black to match her robe. Oaths had been taken, and the gymnasium that had earlier been filled with wanderers and displaced nationals was now full of proud and grateful citizens.

"Welcome, and greetings to our new citizens."

Applause erupted like a cloud bursting over the parched hearts of the people who were longing for a place to call home. We gathered ourselves, and I took mum's hand as we weaved our way through the crowd amidst selfies and self-appointed paparazzi capturing moments of the new naturalization status.

On the ride home, mum sat smiling, reviewing from

time to time the certificate of naturalization. She repeated the last line with the enthusiasm of a child who was announcing a report card full of A's.

"Such person is admitted as a citizen of the United States of America."

"Congratulations, Ma!"

She got so quiet, I wondered if she had slipped into a moment of mental oblivion. Then, as if resuming after a long pause from the earlier conversation, she cleared her throat.

"I'm sorry for all you went through. Try to forget the whole thing."

I turned the words over in my mind. *I'm sorry ... Try to forget the whole thing.* It was both a validation and denial. I wasn't sure if what she was saying was even possible. Could I forget all I'd been through? There may have been times in my life when I wanted to forget, but somewhere along the way, I realized I didn't need to. Everything I had experienced had helped me to become who I am. The baton of individual responsibility may not have been handed to me as it should, but I was still able to pick it up off the ground and run my own leg of the race with it.

It's ironic that now that my mum is dealing with dementia, she finally remembers to say I'm sorry. I didn't need an apology anymore. What happens if you wait your whole life for an apology that you will never get? Waiting for an apology keeps you chained to the offense, and if you don't get one, that's just another grievance to add to the list. Apologies are for those who remain dependent on the actions of others. That no longer described me. I had come to terms with my life, the bumpy parts and the blessed parts. Hearing her apology was nice, but it was more for her benefit than mine.

"Ma, I don't blame you for anything. I'm making sense of my life experiences and my relationships. I'm okay."

That was the closest I ever came to "I forgive you." It was enough for both of us.

In life we are thrust, kicking and screaming, into situations that test our fortitude, our ability to cope, and our willingness to let things go, and sometimes we get wounded in the process. Time does not heal all wounds. That's a fallacy. Depending on the nature and severity of the wound, time alone can cause it to worsen. Over time, what may appear to be a superficial wound can become infected and lead to death if it is not properly treated. In a similar way, a wounded relationship can have devastating consequences if you do not respond to the damage appropriately.

When you have been wounded, you have a right to say "Ouch!" To be denied that right or to repress the expression of the pain creates anger and resentment. If it hurts, it hurts. Say "ouch;" let the tears flow; talk to someone who will listen who is qualified to help you to care for the wound. One of the reasons God gave us emotions and the ability to express them is so that we have an outlet for pain. Keep in mind, however, that the expression of your pain and anger is not the same as healing the wound.

I have yet to see a wound heal just by the wounded person saying "Ouch." It just doesn't happen. It doesn't matter how loudly you say it or how many times, the mere expression of your pain and anger toward the one who hurt you will not bring healing. That expression serves one purpose, which is to let it be known that you have been wounded. But if you want healing, you have to attend to the wound, take whatever precautions you can to protect it from further injury, and apply only those things that will promote healing.

You have limited control over the wounds another person may knowingly or unknowingly try to inflict on you. Trying to control someone else's actions is an exercise in futility. You can set boundaries in place and take precautionary measures, but you cannot stop someone from doing what is in their character, or lack thereof. You can, however, make a distinction between their actions and yours. You can control your own actions and prevent self-inflicted wounds.

One way you can wound yourself is by refusing to let go of the offense, in other words, refusing to forgive. Being unforgiving is like yelling "Ouch!" while at the same time poking your finger into your own wound. You're hurting yourself. Unforgiveness is holding on to the very thing that is causing you pain. If someone drops a lump of hot coal in your hand, the best thing to do is drop the hot coal as soon as possible. Why hold onto it and continue to burn yourself? Let it go. The sooner, the better. You may be able to persuade someone to say that they're sorry, but you can never make them sorry. That's an issue of the heart. Only when you surrender your control of the actions of others will you start to realize the healing power of forgiveness.

Forgiving the one who has wounded you does not mean that you will not remember what they've done to you. You will remember. But when those memories surface, remind yourself that you "dropped the coal." Forgiveness is a process. It is not denying what is wrong but acknowledging and holding on to only what is good for you. If it doesn't help you, you don't need it. It's not about a feeling. It's a decision that you make. At first, you might struggle with forgiving the one who has wounded you because of what they did to you in the past. But as you continue in the process, reminding yourself that you have chosen to forgive and releasing the offense as often as necessary, your heart will be released from pain. What they've done can even become a platform for your progress.

Mum was far from perfect. I could either allow her flaws to distort who I am intended to be or use them as the catalyst for my own spiritual formation and transformation. I choose the latter. If I glance back at her mistakes, it will only be to look for anything beneficial. Otherwise, why bother? That subtle shift in perspective changes everything.

In retrospect, leaving me with my grandparents was one of the greatest gifts my mum ever gave me. Whatever her reasons, she placed me in an environment where I was loved and treasured. Her absence from my life made me appreciate even more the closeness of family. Not being there for me at the crucial stages of my development fueled my desire to make sure I'm there for my girls in theirs. Her devout faith, as obsessive and unbalanced as it seemed, planted the seed for my awareness of the existence and eventual acceptance of God and His involvement in my life. The conflicts in our relationship served as the resistance that built up the muscles of my inner fortitude. I learned how to be strong, and I also learned that I no longer always have to be. I can accept help when I need it. Whatever the circumstance, I have the stamina to buckle down and face it.

Trouble can either make you bitter or better. With God's help and a lot of prayer, I chose the latter. As difficult as it was, I don't regret in the least all that I've done for my mother. I believe God has blessed me for it, not because I wanted to do all that I did, but because I did it even when I didn't want to.

Mum's condition had been declining rapidly, to the point that her doctor told me that I should consider a nursing home.

"Your mom's health is not really going to pan out." He said it as though he'd said those words a thousand times before.

It was getting more difficult to care for her at home. Under the same roof, we were sometimes like unfriendly cats and dogs; best if we stayed away from each other. Her frequent wanderings were precarious, and she needed continuous round the clock care. There was no way I could give her that level of constant attention, not even with the assistance of my husband and children. On most days, my children would be calling me, "Mummy! Mummy!" and my mum would be shouting "Karen! Karen!" right along with them. I felt scattered and torn in so many pieces. I did my best to buy time and just manage as best as I could, but I couldn't avoid the inevitable.

Mum became weakened to the point where therapy became mandatory. I checked her in for three weeks of rehab, and that's when she helped me to make the decision I had been putting off. She was so happy during the time she was there. She was getting physical therapy to help strengthen her body, and she loved all the activity and constant attention from the staff. She had found a different kind of freedom, and she was happier there than being trapped in a room in my home. The decision was made. She would remain at the facility after rehab as a resident of their nursing home.

The day she was moving in, my stomach was in knots. I did everything I could to make her comfortable, but she was more ready for the adjustment than I was. She looked around with a big grin on her face.

"I love it here! God told me this is His plan for me."

And for the first time in my life, I believed without question she had heard from God. It was as if someone had lifted a huge weight off my shoulders. Mum was going to be okay, and that was what I wanted more than anything.

Sometimes the remedy for a relationship is not closeness but distance. I still visit mum four times a week and call her morning and night, mothering her as usual. I can enjoy her better and her me when I'm not stressed by the high demands of caring for her. She's so busy enjoying her new life, she barely has time to call me. I'm the one calling her several times a day to check up on her. Now that we're apart from each other, we're like best friends. She has a different certificate of citizenship in a community of people who can understand and take care of her needs. Mum has a new place to call home, and now we can both finally breathe.

7

MOTHER ISSUES

"If you know what you have, you know what to get rid of." – Julie Morgenstern

Theresa sat across from the therapist's wingback chair. Her skin had started to look as leathery and worn as the settee she sat on. She had started counseling sessions soon after she discovered she had stage four cancer. As I listened to the details of her story, I couldn't help but notice some similarities. It could very well have been me sitting on the other side of that chair.

Theresa grew up in a family that moved and shifted with the tide of whatever bad mood her parents were in.

Her father was a functional addict and a womanizer who appeared as Mr. Charming to everyone except his wife. They fought and argued so much that a normal day seemed out of place.

One day her father got up, dressed, left for work, and never came back. Her mother was never the same after that. She became distant and withdrawn, and depression clouded her ability to handle the responsibilities of raising her children on her own. Theresa, being the oldest at thirteen, had to take care of herself and her six younger siblings. Her mother was cold and distant, as if she blamed her children for her misfortune. She never really interacted except to pour out her brokenness on them with words that projected her own insecurities and self-loathing.

Theresa bore the brunt of the abuse since she was the oldest. She hung around longer than she needed to so that she could act as a buffer between her mother's pain and her younger siblings. By the time she left home, she had vowed never to return. She kept that vow. But when her mother was diagnosed with metastatic breast cancer, none of her siblings were either willing or living close enough to take care of her.

Theresa took her mother in, but she struggled with her decision every day. She fixed her meals, served her, took her to her appointments, bathed her, and cleaned up after her. She did everything for her and resented every minute of it. Over time, her mother, knowing she was at death's door, expressed sorrow for certain things she had done and explained that she didn't know how to communicate with her children or how to really love herself or her kids. Theresa began to realize her mother had a heart after all, but it was too little, too late.

Theresa's mom died, leaving a legacy of conflict between a past she could not change, a present she could not amend, and a future for her child that was still filled with the memories of unresolved issues. Theresa had done her part, taking care of her mother, but bitterness had eaten away at her soul, and cancer was consuming her body. Less than two years later, Theresa followed her mother to the grave.

Coincidence is when God chooses to remain anonymous. Although I was not aware of His influence at the time, I'm convinced that God had something to do with why I chose to be a psychotherapist. I spend a lot of my time listening to people talk about their issues and helping them to find solutions to what they're going through. I worked through many issues resulting from the relationship with my mother which I believe has helped me to develop a level of empathy and compassion for others who are working through their own process of healing and recovery. God has helped and is helping me to break the cycles of my mother's past mistakes. But I still remember a time in the not so distant past when even a particular date on the calendar would trigger a sense of anxiety and inner conflict.

I never used to look forward to Mother's Day. For me, it was nothing to get excited about, and I didn't feel inclined to go above and beyond what I was already doing for my mother. For a long time, it was an annual reminder that the mother-daughter closeness was not there. Mother's Day is a celebration of your mother. But how do you celebrate someone who has been a source or catalyst of so much pain and frustration in your life? The bigger question for me then, and for all of the Theresas in the world, was *why should I care for a parent who didn't really take care of me*? Trying to work through the inner turmoil of answering such a momentous question was a process. The answer started with my under-standing of one word, *honor*. Reconciling the relation-ship with my mother wasn't really about being a dutiful daughter. It was about honoring my mother.

Honor Your Mother

I grew up hearing that I'm supposed to honor my mother and father. My father was not a part of my life, and for the most part, not much of a consideration. But I used to think that honoring my mother meant doing everything in my power to make her happy. I later discovered that is not what it means at all.

Honor is about placing value on who my mother was and is, not based on her actions as a mother but her position. You might be wondering what value you could place on a mother who, like Theresa's, was abusive and detached, or like mine who made most of her decisions based on what was in her own best interest. If you find it difficult to estimate your mother's value, estimate your own value, and the fact that God used her to bring you into this world. Even if your mother was rotten to the core, she delivered you into this world, and that's got to count for something.

Honoring her does not mean that you have to do whatever she wants you to do in order to please her and make her feel happy. It is not your responsibility to make up for any unhappiness in your mother's life. Happiness is a choice, and it's a choice she has to make for herself, just as you have to make that choice for yourself. It is not your responsibility to fill any void in her life or to fulfill her needs. That is a God-sized job.

Maintain Your Boundaries

Boundaries draw the line between behaviors that you will and will not tolerate. One of the most liberating moments in my life was when I realized that it is possible to love my mother and still say 'no' to things she wanted me to do that were detrimental to my wellbeing. It was not easy for me to do at first, but the more I did it, the easier it got.

Toxic behavior is often apparent in the way we communicate. If communication could have cancer, it would be bitterness. Bitterness is what happens when unforgiveness graduates. It is a by-product of anger that has continued for too long. Bitterness rehearses offenses by bringing up the past repeatedly and complains often. Boundaries enable you to say no to bitterness and the behaviors or attitudes that are toxic and contaminate your life, whether those behaviors be your parent's or your own.

Some parents are particularly toxic in their manner of speaking and living. You do not have to allow your mother to hold you hostage to her complaints or let her regurgitate her bitterness until she feels relieved and you feel completely drained or depressed. You can say, "No." Give a respectable warning if you have to, and if the behavior continues, walk away, leave the room, hang up the phone. Do whatever you have to do to keep from getting contaminated. Your life is not your mother's dumping-ground. She may not understand or like your 'no,' but she can learn to respect it and live with it.

Understand Your Responsibility

One needs to know the difference between privilege and responsibility. Take financial support, for example. There is a difference between being a provider and providing financial support. It is the responsibility of parents to make financial provision and leave an inheritance for their children. This does not mean that you should blame your parents for what you don't have. This also does not mean that if your mother needs assistance, you should not help her, especially if she is a widow or has no other help. If you are blessed to be in a position to help with her financial needs and reasonable wants, keep your boundaries intact, and consider doing so. However, you are not responsible for bailing your mother out of poor financial decisions, especially if it is habitual.

One of the things you are responsible for is to love your mother. When I use the word 'love,' I'm not referring to an emotional feeling or the expression of any such feeling. When I speak of love, I'm speaking of

God's kind of love, which means *doing what is in the best interest of another with no expectation of return.* If I based my love for my mother on my feelings or in response to some of the things she did or did not do in the past, it might have been difficult to truly love her. But knowing God loves me in spite of and in light of all my imperfectness, and because He has put His love in my heart, He has made me capable of loving her. So, I choose to love her. That allows me to realize the potential of all I am capable of being.

When your love is not predicated on your feelings or what she does or doesn't do, you will embrace peace for yourself. As long as you hold on to the expectations of what your mother should have done or what she should have said, as long as you keep expecting her to become that loving, supportive, nurturing mother you had always hoped she would be, you set yourself up for disappointment, anger, resentment, and bitterness.

I'm not suggesting you rule out the possibility that she can become that person if she is still alive. With God, all things are possible. But you may need to face the reality that she may never become that person. You have to ask yourself the hard question, *what if she never changes?* Her change is outside the domain of your control. However, you can decide that even if your mother never changes for the better, you will.

Give Freely

Some mothers specialize in emotional manipulation. They are experts in making their children feel guilty in order to get them to do what they want them to do. You may have fallen prey to this kind of manipulation and have spent your life giving to mom out of a sense of guilt or obligation. The result many times is built-up resentment, anger, and bitterness. Giving should be done without reluctance or feeling forced—freely, cheerfully, and readily. If this is not how you feel when you give, check to see if your boundary line is being crossed or if there is some underlying offense. This brings me to my next and final point.

Forgive

I've said a lot about forgiveness in the previous chapter. But I cannot end this book without giving a final word about forgiveness. For many of you, forgiving your mother is your day-to-day struggle. You must forgive her, not because she deserves or asks for it, or says she's sorry. She may never admit the things she's done wrong. She may not even remember them. Forgive mom because God has forgiven you.

Remember, forgiveness is a decision you make; it's

not a feeling. When you don't forgive, you carry the weight of the offense. Your mother may have all kinds of issues for various reasons, but why should you carry the weight of *her* issues? Refuse to remain in the womb of your mother's issues. Forgive and cut the umbilical cord that has been nourishing you from the placenta of her bitterness and unhappiness. Mom may have had issues, but they no longer have to be yours.

NOTES

In this section, I have included a list of scripture references that were discussed in the closing chapter. I trust that they will help you in your process of making peace with your parent.

Honor Your Parents

Ephesians 6:2 AMPC Honor (esteem and value as precious) your father and your mother—this is the first commandment with a promise.

Maintain Your Boundaries

2 Corinthians 7:1 AMPC Therefore, since these [great] promises are ours, beloved, let us cleanse ourselves from everything that contaminates and defiles body and spirit, and bring [our] consecration to completeness in the [reverential] fear of God.

Understand Your Responsibility

Proverbs 13:22a NIRV A good person leaves what they own to their children and grandchildren.

1 Timothy 5:3-4 AMPC [Always] treat with great consideration and give aid to those who are truly widowed (solitary and without support). But if a widow has children or grandchildren, see to it that these are first made to understand that it is their religious duty [to defray their natural obligation to those] at home, and make return to their parents or grandparents [for all their care by contributing to their maintenance], for this is acceptable in the sight of God.

Romans 5:5 AMPC God's love has been poured out in our hearts through the Holy Spirit Who has been given to us.

Give Freely

2 Corinthians 9:7 AMPC Let each one [give] as he has made up his own mind and purposed in his heart, not reluctantly or sorrowfully or under compulsion, for God loves (He takes pleasure in, prizes above other things, and is unwilling to abandon or to do without) a cheerful (joyous, "prompt to do it") giver [whose heart is in his giving].

Forgive

Ephesians 4:32 AMPC And become useful and helpful and kind to one another, tenderhearted (compassionate, understanding, loving-hearted), forgiving one another [readily and freely], as God in Christ forgave you.

ACKNOWLEDGMENTS

Thanks to my beautiful girls for showering me with affection and bringing out the best in me as a mother. Mummy loves you!

Heartfelt thanks to Aleathea Dupree for believing there was a book in me and helping to bring it out. You made writing a book with such difficult subject matter an enjoyable experience.

A very special thanks to my "White Socks" for taking my mother as your own, always being there for me, and never complaining no matter how many times your sleep was interrupted. You are the answer to my prayers and the proof that God cares about the details of my life. (Do you believe I wrote a book now?)

And to my mum, thank you for having the courage to bring me into a world that brought you so much pain.

ABOUT THE AUTHOR

Karen Oke is a Psychotherapist and Christian Life Coach. She is passionate about helping people begin their process of change to improve their life's circumstances. Karen lives in Texas with her husband and children.

Connect with the author at
www.karenokebooks.com

Printed in Great Britain
by Amazon

37640794R00056